KIMBERLY JANNICE BREWER

Bipolar Unraveled

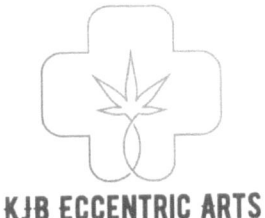

KJB ECCENTRIC ARTS

First published by KJB Eccentric Arts 2022

Copyright © 2022 by Kimberly Jannice Brewer

Kimberly Jannice Brewer asserts the moral right to be identified as the author of this work.

Kimberly Jannice Brewer has no responsibility for the persistence or accuracy of URLs for external or third-party Internet Websites referred to in this publication and does not guarantee that any content on such Websites is, or will remain, accurate or appropriate.

Designations used by companies to distinguish their products are often claimed as trademarks. All brand names and product names used in this book and on its cover are trade names, service marks, trademarks and registered trademarks of their respective owners. The publishers and the book are not associated with any product or vendor mentioned in this book. None of the companies referenced within the book have endorsed the book.

First edition

This book was professionally typeset on Reedsy. Find out more at reedsy.com

Contents

1	Bipolar Introduction	1
2	Bipolar Disorder	4
3	Risk Factors	8
4	Bipolar Disorder Summarized	13
5	Subtypes of Bipolar Disorder	18
6	Treatment of Bipolar Disorder	21
7	Medications for Bipolar Disorder	23
8	Medications for Depression	27
9	Medication Side Effects	33
10	Bipolar Disorder Effects	35
11	Managing a Mental Illness	41
12	Comorbidity	45
13	References	48
	About the Author	52

One

Bipolar Introduction

Search the web...

I entered bipolar disorder and about 91,200,000 results pop up... probably more since that day.

How many can I relate to completely?

0. Zero. Nada. Nothing. None of them.

I'm not sure if it's because the idea of spreading mental health awareness is simply stating what the symptoms and treatments are for these mood disorders.... But the public just reads that. Brochures and pamphlets are about as much information people receive about their illnesses.

Those diagnosed with mood disorders need a separate private

server of some kind, where they have free access to all the research data available about their illness. I had access when I was attending my universities, but after graduating the access wears off as time goes on. Then you have to pay to gain access to data related to you? It's almost as much as asking permission to enter your house but paying a fee before entering even though you are welcome. I suppose that is the way everything is now, monetized. Not me though, I am searching for all the information I can and writing about it for others to read freely.

Then Google says that "people" ask: What are 5 signs of bipolar? What are the types of bipolar? What is the personality of a bipolar person? *(This one made me laugh out loud)* Can a bipolar person live a normal life? *LOL!*

All of these here, I feel are questions of people wondering if they have anything similar to what they saw on a TikTok, YouTube, or Twitter video and wondering if they looked it up like a horoscope that they'd be able to determine if they had a mood disorder or not? It does not work that way, however, if you do find yourself feeling different and asking these questions gets you closer to something you relate to, then please seek professional help from a licensed counselor or therapist, or just talk to your health practitioner. If you do not have one and require immediate help, please refer to **Mental Health Help.**

My Setting

From the eyes, head, and hands, who feels the ins and outs of bipolar disorder. I want to share knowledge. Here it is first-hand.

Bipolar Introduction

My information will include first-hand experiences, knowledge, and medical information on what is bipolar disorder and possible treatments.

I want to become a part of the knowledge that can help me be a guide for those suffering from bipolar disorder. If you read this, I just hope you come to an understanding that we may not one hundred percent connect, we won't be alike in everything, but you're not alone in the war. Your battle matters.

I do not have a support network. However, I hope this provides a stepping stone to a better support system for myself. And writing about it may be able to help you set your own up. Remember, this is about you. Maybe you want to share this material with someone you know to better understand this world of ours.

Bipolar disorder is a scary set of words that have been used throughout thriller and psychological movies, openly thrown out there when someone seems to be normal then shifts to an angry outburst or sad depressive mode, they're being "bipolar"... the act of being bipolar is not something that exists...making the statement false. Bipolar disorder is a mood disorder, it is more than just a diagnosis that can be dealt with, with medication or not. I have done both. I have lived with this disorder for over 20 years, it has had everything to do with all the choices and paths I have chosen throughout my life. I am a person who has and will always have a brain illness and I try to live a *normal* (*haha*), happy, content life.

Two

Bipolar Disorder

Bipolar Disorder

Bipolar Disorder, also known as manic depression or manic-depressive illness, is a psychiatric disorder, a brain disorder that causes unusual shifts in mood, energy and activity levels, and the challenge of carrying everyday tasks. This mood disorder is a mental illness, a disease that affects the brain. This condition is a serious lifelong challenge.

"Psychiatrists and psychologists usually think of bipolar disorder as a set of symptoms, which must be present in clusters (that is, more than one at a time) and last for a certain length of time, usually in "episodes" that have a beginning phase, a phase in which symptoms are at their worst, and a recovery phase" (Miklowitz, 2019).

Then, people who know the person may have a different perspective and it may refer to a family member or friend viewing the person's personality, or describing their behaviors as erratic and "moody". While people with the illness often see bipolar disorder as a secondary approach to their different life experiences of their ups and downs.

More than 5.7 million American adults have bipolar disorder, not including worldwide and those who have yet to be diagnosed. Bipolar disorder typically starts in late adolescence or early adulthood, although children and older adults can also suffer from this condition. This condition is a treatable disease that can be helped to improve behavior, feelings, and moods. This condition affects parts of the brain that control emotion, thought, and drive and the causes for this may be a complex set of genetic and environmental factors.

Bipolar disorder is a brain disease. This condition affects areas of the brain through imbalances of brain chemicals in the areas of the brain that help human beings regulate emotion, thinking processes, and energy levels. Mostly, bipolar disorder happens when someone experiences a stressful event such as job loss, family argument, a serious relationship problem, or even a simple triggering event can send an individual to spiral through their imbalances. Scientists have yet to pinpoint the true cause behind bipolar disorder, but they do know that the illness is inherited. Bipolar disorder is considered a bio-psycho-social illness, some factors such as genetics cannot be controlled, but other factors that may worsen bipolar disorder, like a stressful and overly tasked-filled job, can be changed.

Traumas can also be risk factors for increasing the risk of developing bipolar disorder. At least half of the cases of bipolar disorder develop before the age of 25. This condition develops among teenagers or in early adulthood. Bipolar disorder is not very easy to spot, even then, the symptoms may be viewed as separate problems, treated separately, while they are parts of a bigger problem. Many people suffer for years before committing to getting treated, then the hurdle of getting the correct diagnosis is the beginning, the ups and downs and trials of medications are a long journey as this is a long-term illness that needs management throughout a person's life.

> Furthermore, researchers have learned that the brain structure and function of people with bipolar disorder versus those who do not have bipolar disorder or have other psychiatric illnesses; are different. There is no known cause for bipolar disorder but some people are born with genes for this disorder, however, the likelihood of developing it is not guaranteed. Also, the ability to develop or have developed better coping skills or a way of handling stress places a role in the development of bipolar disorder symptoms. It is very helpful to learn coping skills, even remembering the basic one, *"breathe in through your nose, exhale through your mouth"*. Sometimes, drug abuse such as the use of alcohol, amphetamines, cocaine, etc., can trigger this disorder.

Brain-imaging studies are helping scientists learn what goes wrong in the brain to produce bipolar disorder and other mental illnesses. New brain-imaging techniques allow researchers to take pictures of the living brain at work, to examine its structure and activity, without the need for surgery or other invasive procedures. These techniques include magnetic resonance imaging (MRI), positron emission tomography (PET), and functional magnetic resonance imaging (fMRI). There is evidence from imaging studies that the brains of people with bipolar disorder may differ from the brains of healthy individuals. As the differences are more clearly identified and defined through research, scientists will gain a better understanding of the underlying causes of the illness, and eventually may be able to predict which types of treatment will work most effectively.

Three

Risk Factors

Risk factors for bipolar disorder

There is no single cause for bipolar disorder. Scientists are still learning about the possible causes of this disorder, but many factors act together and contribute to producing this illness or increasing the risk of developing bipolar disorder.

It is one of several conditions referred to as mood disorders, which are diagnosed based on the occurrence of episodes. Okay, well what is an episode? An episode is caused by a mood disorder, it refers to a set of symptoms that occur during the same period.

Risk Factors

What Is a Bipolar Mood Episode?

- A set of symptoms that go together, with a beginning prodromal phase, a middle acute phase, and a final recovery phase.
- The polarity of a mood episode can be depressed, manic, hypomanic, or mixed.
- Episodes can last anywhere from a few days to several months.
- Some people switch polarities in the middle of an episode (for example, from depressed to manic or from manic to mixed). (Miklowitz, 2019)

What kind of symptoms?
That's where I think it is complicated because individuals vary from person to person. Individuals with this mood disorder experience manic or hypomanic episodes (intense feeling of euphoria), depressive episodes (intense low periods more than just sad), and potentially some psychotic symptoms during these stages. Throw all of those together into a shaker bottle, don't forget the metal ball thingy, and you get mixed episodes.

Everyone with bipolar disorder has different variations in their moods, I have yet to find someone alike. What about periods when there aren't any symptoms, that's what they like to call periods of euthymia or periods or "normalcy" whatever that is. And for those who constantly vary from mood to mood, that means they are cycling. Not on purpose for exercise or anything, just because the brain tells them to cycle back and forth from super manic to depressed and mixed moods.

What's different from everyday people's mood variations?

The difference is other people do not feel the intense and distressing symptoms that are mental, emotional, and physical either during a depressive episode or a manic/hypomanic episode to where it pushes individuals out of reality. The swings in moods are intense, distressing, and very overwhelming. The intensity of bipolar disorder symptoms reminds me of an oscilloscope, up and down…. some people's graphs are more up than down, and some more down than up, but these are only the intense parts of a rollercoaster; people without this mood disorder have periods where the rollercoaster coasts; people with this mood disorder are always in the scariest highest point or the scariest drop of their lives. How exhausting!

The following are risk factors that may increase the chances of becoming ill or having an episode:

- Life changes (positive or negative stress): loss of a job, beginning or ending a relationship, and the birth of a child
- Alcohol and drug abuse: drinking binges; experimenting with illegal drugs; excessive marijuana use or opiate use
- Sleep deprivation: changing time zones; cramming for exams; sudden changes in sleep-wake habits
- Family distress or interpersonal conflicts: High levels of criticism from a parent, spouse, or partner; provocative or hostile environments with family members or coworkers
- Inconsistency with medications: Suddenly stopping your

Risk Factors

mood stabilizers; regularly missing dosages

The following are protective factors that decrease the chances of having an episode:

- Observing and monitoring your moods and fluctuation triggers: Keep a **daily mood journal** or a **social rhythm chart**.
- Exercise: Jogging, yoga, long walks, gym workouts, hiking, biking
- Maintaining regular daily and nightly routines: Going to bed and waking up at regular hours; having a predictable exercise and social schedule
- Relying on social and family supports: Clear communication with relatives; asking your significant others for help in emergencies
- Engaging in regular medical and psychosocial treatment: Staying on a consistent medication regimen, obtaining weekly psychotherapy; attending support groups

Cool! A list of things I have already gone over a million times, right? It is always difficult to try to implement any of these strategies to maintain your health. However, implementing one or two will help to control swinging into severe mood episodes.

Maintaining a **mood chart** will help to keep track of activity levels for yourself, for your doctor, and it can also help identify extra triggers in specific environment settings. Each chart allows you to track moods each day for up to a month. A few minutes before you brush your teeth, take the time to chart your moods. Keeping the charted moods each month will help you to guide you throughout the year. The more you do it, the better you can point out and examine what it is that creates your bipolar disorder shifts. It can be difficult to remember to chart but doing it at a certain time day to day will help you keep up with it. That's a huge accomplishment for your mental health.

Four

Bipolar Disorder Summarized

The highs

Everyone hears about the highs of bipolar disorder, this is called mania. Many people experience mania as a highly elevated mood, mentally and/or physically where it can noticeably cause a disturbance in the individual's mood. This includes elation, becoming irritable or expansive: that is thinking in a euphoric state of mind with delusions of grandiosity. Mania is more than just feeling like you have a zap of energy and all of sudden remember to do Spring cleaning in October. It is more than just feeling great about yourself and being confident that everything will be okay, it supersedes all those feelings because all of the moods become intense and very heightened. With this rollercoaster trip the symptoms include a variety of these:

- Increased energy
- Racing thoughts or flight of ideas
- Inflated self-esteem
- A decreased need for sleep
- Abnormal irritability
- Extreme happiness
- Poor judgment
- Overparticipation in risky activities
- Excessive talking or pressured speech
- Clear evidence of distractibility
- Increased level of goal-focused activity at home, at work or sexually
- Excessive pleasurable activities, often with painful consequences

All of these symptoms need to be active during at least one week to be considered mania or longer. The mood disturbance is enough to cause impairment at work or danger to the self or others. The initial symptoms of mania oncoming are pleasurable, many people with bipolar disorder look forward to going into a manic episode due to the pleasurable effects, and getting out of a depressive state. Also, the mood must not be a result of substance abuse or another medical condition. Mania may cause negative financial, career, or relationship consequences. Often mania leads to problems so severe that a person must be hospitalized.

However, not all mania episodes result in hospitalization, but it may cause great turmoil in a person's life during those days of mania. When individuals experience mania, they may also have auditory or visual hallucinations, which are usually only present during manic phases. Some of the most common delusions are delusions of paranoia, in which patients believe that people are stalking, targeting, or surveilling them. Usually, there is poor insight during psychosis and delusions are not noticed by the individual; the issue is often noticed by others, family members, friends, co-workers, or even strangers or the police.

Besides mania, there is also hypomania. Hypomania involves having the same symptoms as above, however, they are different in severity the strength of the symptoms. That is, hypomanic episodes may not cause impairment in social or occupational situations; does not pose a danger to the individual or others. According to the DSM-5, hypomanic episodes must last three days or more. A hypomanic phase can be coupled with full manic episodes or it can occur at the beginning or at the end of severe depression. That is why many bipolar people look forward to it, however, it may also be a sign that a more severe manic episode is on the way or it may be a sign that a person's roller coaster is going to go off the rails and crash, becoming depressed.

There is a common mnemonic "DIG FAST" that is used to aid clinicians in remembering to ask, however, I feel it should be helpful to all of those affected by any type of bipolar disorder.

- D: Distractibility
- I: Irresponsibility/Irritability
- G: Grandiosity
- F: Flight of Ideas
- A: Activity increases
- S: Sleep less

- T: Talkativeness intensifies

The evaluation must include the full DSM-5 criteria as mentioned above and the individual's abrupt change in mood that lasts at least one week (Stahl, Morrissette; 2019).

The lows

Depression is not only severe sadness. Depression is more serious than just a word, it is a medical condition that people with bipolar disorder experience. It is more than just a bad day at work or just a sad mood when you have had a crummy day at work or school. Major depression is a medical disorder that lasts at least two weeks. During those two weeks or longer, physical and emotional symptoms make it very difficult to function in life. According to the DSM-5, the person must experience five symptoms with one symptom being either a depressed mood or a loss of pleasure or interest (with the possibility of experiencing both).

Clinical depression is experiencing the loss of pleasure in activities that used to be fun or exciting. The symptoms of depression may include the following:

- Feelings of sadness
- Hopelessness or excessive guilt
- Pessimism
- Difficulty sleeping; hypersomnia (oversleeping) or insomnia
- Poor concentration and memory
- Low energy or fatigue

- Change in appetite; with a significant change in loss or increase in appetite
- Psychomotor agitation or retardation (agitation: a series if unintentional and purposeless motions that stem from mental tension and anxiety for an individual; retardation: motor and cognitive impairments including slowness)
- Preoccupied with death or suicide; person has a plan or has attempted suicide

Depression changes the way a person interprets and thinks of the world. For instance, it is not uncommon for people who are severely depressed to feel helpless and hopeless that suicide may be the only rational alternative to their current situation. It is important to remember that depression is treatable, with time.

Be patient with yourself if you are on the raw end of the depression. You give others many chances or you let others have opportunities to do better for themselves when with you, why not give yourself the same patience?

Five

Subtypes of Bipolar Disorder

What does this mean? It means there is more than just one type of bipolar disorder, there are four types according to the DSM-5:

- Bipolar disorder type one
- Bipolar disorder type two
- Cyclothymic disorder
- Other specified bipolar and other disorders (used to be known as bipolar not otherwise specified)

Bipolar Disorder Type One

Bipolar disorder type one (Bipolar I) is the mood disorder of experiencing states of depression and mania, also, this is probably one of the more traditional forms of bipolar disorder. Bipolar I is a mood disorder in which the individual has experienced one or more episodes of mania. It is not necessary for an individual to experience an episode of depression to get a diagnosis of Bipolar I, however, most people who have Bipolar I experience episodes of both mania and depression. Most individuals with Bipolar I will have episodes of both depression and mania, while a few individuals will have episodes of mania alone.

Bipolar Disorder Type Two

Bipolar disorder type two (Bipolar II) is a mood disorder where individuals experience at least one hypomanic episode but never a full-blown manic episode. In order to meet the criteria for Bipolar II, an individual must also have had at least one episode of depression. People with Bipolar II do not experience psychosis. However, it is not considered any less serious than Bipolar I.

Cyclothymic Disorder

Cyclothymic disorder is considered a less severe version of bipolar disorder. There are periods of chronic mood instability (one year for children or adolescents, two years for adults); during this period individuals experience abnormal mood states that may seem elevated and low states, however, they do not meet the full criteria for mania, hypomania, or depression.

Other Specified Bipolar and Other Disorder [Bipolar Not Otherwise Specified]

Bipolar NOS is periods of abnormal mood elevation, this diagnosis is included in the DSM-5 to summarize the version of bipolar disorder that does not meet the criteria for any other subtypes of bipolar disorder. Symptoms may have been too brief or too few to meet the criteria for any subtypes, sometimes it is referred to as Atypical bipolar disorder.

Six

Treatment of Bipolar Disorder

Bipolar disorder is one of the mental health illnesses that cannot be cured, however, it can be treated and managed. However, much like any other illness like hypothyroidism or diabetes, different medications affect people differently, and different therapies or treatments are adjusted for each individual. The key is to know how to be successful for yourself, and your own well-being, and not base it on others' experiences of their illness.

The medication selected by your doctor to treat bipolar disorder will depend on the mood you are in at the time (i.e., manic, hypomanic, depressed, or mixed), and/or the presence of psychosis, or any other concurrent illnesses like anxiety, obsessive-compulsive disorder, etc. Other factors such as other diseases or other present medications should be made aware of to know if there will be any interaction or counter interaction.

Seven

Medications for Bipolar Disorder

[Medication (Brand name:): common side effects; may interact with-]

There are thirteen approved medications by the Food and Drug Administration (FDA) that can be used to treat bipolar disorder - each for different mood states.

- Aripiprazole (*Abilify*): **Insomnia, nausea, restlessness, tiredness;** *antidepressants such as Prozac or Paxil, Mood stabilizers such as Equetro or Tegretol*
- Asenapine (*Saphris*): **Sleepiness, dizziness, strange sense of taste, numbing of the mouth, nausea, increased appetite, feeling tired, weight gain;** *Antihypertensive medications, antidepressants, anxiety medications*

- Carbamazepine, extended released capsules (*Equetro*): **Dizziness, drowsiness, nausea, dry mouth, blurred vision, decreased white blood cell count, can rarely cause severe skin rashes;** *birth control pills-making them ineffective, mood stabilizers such as Lithium, Lamictal, or Depakote, Anticonvulsant medications, Anxiety medications, macrolife, antibiotics, tricyclic antidepressants, cancer medications, HIV/AIDS medications, cytotoxic or immunosuppressive*
- Cariprazine (*Vraylar*): **Muscle stiffness, indigestion, vomiting, sleepiness, restlessness;** *antidepressants, pain medications, anxiety medications, mood stabilizers such as lithium, anticonvulsants such as Lamictal, antipsychotics such as Latuda or Seroquel*
- Divalproex Sodium (*Depakote*): **Nausea, shaking, weight gain, decrease in blood platelets, rash, pancreatitis, liver dysfunction (rare), polycystic ovary syndrome (rare);** *aspirin or other blood thinning medications, mood stabilizers such as Equetro, Tegretol, or Lamictal, Barbiturates, Cyclosporine (Neoral or Sandimmune)*
- Fluoxetine + Olanzapine (*Symbyax*): **Dizziness, drowsiness, dehydration, headache, nausea, sweating;** *MAOI antidepressants, antipsychotics such as Mellarl, pain medications, sleep medications, blood pressure or heart medications, anticonvulsants, herbal supplements, alcohol*
- Lamotrigine (*Lamictal*): **Sleepiness, blurred vision, sensitivity to sunlight, headache, nausea, can rarely cause severe skin rashes;** Mood stabilizers such as Depakote, Equetro, or Tegretol, Antibiotics such as Bactrim, Septra, or Proloprim, anticonvulsants, birth control pills, barbiturates
- Lithium carbonate (*Lithionate, Lithotabs, Lithobid, Eskalith*):

Medications for Bipolar Disorder

Shaking, nausea, increased thirst/dry mouth, frequent urination, diarrhea, fatigue/dull feeling, lowered thyroid activity, weight gain, kidney trouble, avoid sweating too much or getting dehydrated, which can make your blood lithium levels toxic; *birth control pills, antidepressants, pain medications, anxiety medications, caffeine, mood stabilizers such as Equetro or Tegretol, anticonvulsants such as Dilantin, antibacterial medications such as Flagyl, iodine, heart, blood pressure, or diuretic medications*

- Olanzapine (*Zyprexa*): **Drowsiness, dry mouth, shaking, increased appetite, weight gain;** *anxiety medications, sleep medications*
- Quetiapine fumarate (*Seroquel*): **weight gain, dry mouth, constipation; stiness/restlessness, shaking, sedation, low blood pressure;** *barbiturates, antibiotics or antifungal medications, anxiety medications, stomach medications such as Tagamet, steroid medications, alcohol*
- Risperidone (*Risperdal*): **weight gain, sedation, increased saliva, stiness/restlessness, shaking, low blood pressure;** *blood pressure or heart medications, antipsychotics, anxiety medications, Parkinson medications*
- Ziprasidone (*Geodon*): **stiness/restlessness, nausea/dizziness, insomnia, tiredness, cough, upset stomach, shaking, rash, tell your doctor if you have ever had heart problems. Contact your doctor or an emergency room immediately if you faint or feel a change in your heartbeat;** *heart and blood pressure medications, cytotoxic or immunosuppressive medications, anticonvulsants, anxiety or sleep medications, Parkinson medications, antibiotic or antibacterial medications, antipsychotics, medications used after surgery, malaria*

Bipolar Unraveled

medications, mood stabilizers, MAOI antidepressants

Eight

Medications for Depression

Medications approved by the FDA for treating Depression (not specifically for bipolar disorder)

[**Medication class**-Medication (*Brand name*): **common side effects;** *may interact with-*]

- **Selective serotonin reuptake inhibitors (SSRI)**- Citalopram, escitalopram, fluvoxamine, paroxetine, sertraline, vilazodone HCI (*Celexa, Lexapro, Luvox, Paxil, Prozac, Zoloft, Vibryd*): **nausea, insomnia, sleepiness, agitation, sexual dysfunction;** *MAOI antidepressants, tricyclic antidepressants, alcohol, anxiety medications, blood thinning medications, anticonvulsants, heart medications*
- **Norepinephrine and dopamine reuptake inhibitors**

(NDRI) - Bupropion (Wellbutrin): **agitation, insomnia, anxiety, dry mouth, headache, seizures are a danger when there are specific risk factors such as previous seizures, heart trauma, eating disorders, or abrupt stopping of alcohol, anxiety medications, or sleep;** *MAOI antidepressants, tricyclic antidepressants, anxiety medications, steroid medications, anticonvulsants, alcohol, diabetes medications*

- Serotonin antagonist and reuptake inhibitor (SARI)- Trazodone, Nefazodone (*Desyrel*): **nausea, dizziness, sleepiness, dry mouth, constipation, weight gain, Nefazodone can rarely cause serious liver damage;** *Anxiety medications such as BuSpar or Ativan, MAOI antidepressants, Heart medications such as Lanoxin or Digitek, sleep medications*
- Serotonin and norepinephrine reuptake inhibitor (SNRI) - Venlafaxin, Duloxetine, Levomilnacipran (*Effexor, Cymbalta, Fetzima*): **anxiety, nausea, dizziness, sleepiness, sexual dysfunction, withdrawal symptoms when stopped abruptly;** *MAOI antidepressants, stomach medications such as Tagamet*

- Noradrenergic and specific serotonergic antidepressant (NaSSA) - Clomipramine, amitriptyli (*Anafranil, Elavil*): **sleepiness, increased appetite, weight gain, dizziness, dry mouth, constipation;** *MAOI antidepressants, alcohol, anxiety medications*
- Tricyclic (TCA) Tetracyclic - Clomipramine, Amitriptyline, Desipramine, Nortriptyline, Imipramine, Protriptyline,

Medications for Depression

Amoxapine, Maprotiline (*Anafranil, Elavil, Norpramin, Pamelor, Surmontil, Tofranil, Vivactil, Asendin, Ludiomil*): **sleepiness, increased appetite, weight gain, dizziness, dry mouth, constipation, urinary retention, increased appetite, weight gain, low blood pressure, sexual dysfunction, may be toxic if levels in blood get too high;** *Alcohol, sleep medications, allergy medications, cold medications, pain medications, heart medications, anxiety medications, birth control pills, anticonvulsants, spasm or cramp medications*

- **Monoamine oxidase inhibitor (MAOI)** - Phenelzine, Tranylcpromine, Isocarboxazid, Selegiline (*Nardil, Parnate, Marplan, Emsam):* **dizziness, dry mouth, urinary retention, sleep problems, low blood pressure, weight gain, sexual dysfunction, can cause dangerously high blood pressure if taken with the wrong food;** *Fatal interaction with some prescribed and over-the-counter medications including pain or cold medications, foods containing tyramine, such as some cheeses, meats, or beans, caffeine, alcohol*

Anticonvulsants that may be prescribed for Bipolar Disorder

(but not officially approved for this use)

[Medication (*Brand name*): **common side effects;** *may interact with-*]

- Carbamazepine (*Equetro, Tegretol, Tegretol-XR, Epitol, Carbatrol):* **blurred vision, dizziness, dry mouth, drowsiness,**

nausea, decreased white blood cell, shaking, if rash occurs contact your doctor immediately; *birth control pills (can make them ineffective), mood stabilizers such as Lithium, Depakote, or Lamictal, Tricyclic antidepressants, other anticonvulsants, macrolide antibiotics, anxiety medications, cancer medications, HIV-AIDS medications, Cytotoxic or immunosuppressive medications, grapefruit juice*

- Oxcarbazepine *(Trileptal)* : **blurred vision, dizziness, dry mouth, sedation, upset stomach, drowsiness, unsteadiness;** *drugs that interact with carbamazepine (see above), birth control pills, blood pressure or heart medications*
- Topiramate *(Topomax)*: **drowsiness, memory problems, feeling "dulled", weight loss, kidney stones, if you have changes in vision, eye pain, or redness, or increased eye pressure, contact your doctor immediately;** *birth control pills, other anticonvulsants, motion sickness or glaucoma medications such as Diamox, heart medications, sleep medications, allergy medications, alcohol, tobacco*
- Zonisamide *(Zonegran)*: **possible allergic reaction, drowsiness, upset stomach, headache, irritability, inability to sweat (contact your doctor if you get overheated or feverish);** *birth control pills, other anticonvulsants, SSRI antidepressants, antibiotic or antifungal medications, allergy medications, heart medications, alcohol*

Please note that these lists may not include all possible side effects or all possible interactions. You should thoroughly discuss all medication choices with your doctor. Research and look up information on the medication, know what it may be like, and whether it is the right one or the correct ones

Medications for Depression

prescribed to you.

Depression and Bipolar Support Alliance (DBSA) does not endorse or recommend the use of any specific treatment or medication for mood disorders. Consult your doctor for more information about specific treatments or medications. Some of the uses under discussion in this brochure may not have been approved by the FDA. (DBSA, n.d.).

Severe manic or mixed mood, typical medications that are prescribed include:

- *Antipsychotics* - a class of medications that are used whether or not psychosis is present. These medications include quetiapine (Seroquel) and olanzapine (Zyprexa), among others.
- *Valproate (Depakote)* - an anticonvulsant that was originally used to treat seizure disorders but now is also used as a mood stabilizer in bipolar disorder.
- *Lithium* - a mood stabilizing drug.

In severe cases, a mood stabilizing drug (i.e., lithium or valproate) can be combined with an antipsychotic.

When **mania is not severe** or **mixed mood**, is **hypomanic**, the following medications are used:

- Lithium
- Valproate or carbamazepine (Tegretol)
- An antipsychotic such as aripiprazole (Abilify) or olanzap-

ine (Zyprexa)

When **depressed phase** of bipolar disorder is present, the top choices for medications include:

- Quetiapine (Seroquel) - an antipsychotic that can stabilize mood.
- Lamotrigine (Lamictal) - an anticonvulsant that was originally used to treat seizure disorders but now is also used as a mood stabilizer in bipolar disorder.
- Lithium

Nine

Medication Side Effects

Bipolar Medication Side Effects

Any medications bring about side effects and risks of developing while treating your mood disorder. However, your doctor will select a medicine or a medication for you because they feel that its benefits are higher than the risks associated with the medicine. Some people experience many side effects, while some people experience none. Side effects are usually at their worst at the beginning of any bipolar medication, but they reduce or go away as treatment is continued. For me, it has been at the very beginning that lasts for two weeks, and every so often it cycles where some side effects like nausea, increased thirst, fatigue, for example, come back while on my medications, but it settles.

If you are ever concerned about side effects from any medication or medication interactions, talk to your doctor right away to adjust the dose, change medications, or help you in some other form. There are many other options!

It is important to know what is the proper dosage and the side effects that may potentially affect you.

Do I need medications?

There will always be mixed feelings about taking medications, and really, even thinking of taking something for a headache, most people choose not to do so. However, many studies have shown that medications can provide benefits for people with episodes of depression and mania. Medications can aid in preventing these episodes from occurring, they are a tool to help you feel better and take charge of your life.

Medications will not cure bipolar disorder, but they will help provide you with a better sense of control over your mood swings and any other related symptoms. However, it is important to know what medications you are on, what they do or may possibly do, and how they can help you on short term and long term issues.

Ten

Bipolar Disorder Effects

What happens to you because of bipolar disorder? Not just the medication side effects, but the effects of having this mental illness as a part of your personal being?

Memory

> "Little is known about the physiology of memory storage in the brain. Some researchers suggest that memories are stored at specific sites, and others say that memories involve widespread brain regions working together; both processes may in fact be involved" (Nishiyama et al., 1998). There are many brain structures that are involved in the

> process of memory, they include the hippocampus, hypothalamus, thalamus, and temporal lobes. If there is damage to any one of them, this can cause memory problems. When a person has trouble remembering something, it is generally not the fault of the entire memory system—just an inefficient component in the memory system (Nishiyama et al., 1998).

Let's take a look at **Norepinephrine**, a neurotransmitter associated with stress also appears to be linked to memories (especially memories associated with stress). When there are low levels of norepinephrine, bipolar disorder reacts to a depressive episode, in contrast, with high levels of norepinephrine, the manic phase of bipolar disorder occurs. Bipolar disorder medications affect norepinephrine, and it is important to discuss this with your doctor as medications may need to be changed or adjusted.

First, it is well-known that several psychotropic agents—especially anticholinergic medication (Nishiyama et al., 1998) and benzodiazepines (Rammsayer et al., 2000; Tonne et al., 1995)—decrease neurocognitive functioning in some patients. Cognitive deficits should by no means be regarded as tolerable side effects of psychopharmacological intervention, as they may endanger medication compliance and often reduce the already compromised cognitive resources of patients, thereby enhancing the patients' vulnerability to stress and renewed psychosis. For future research, new treatment options need to be tested that may offer surplus effects on neurocognition.

Additionally, another study analyzed the influences of antipsychotic treatment and "relapse" on brain volume among those with schizophrenia. For the study, they analyzed 202 patients who had undergone MRI scans over an average of 7 years. The researchers pointed out that the greater the intensity of antipsychotic treatment, the smaller the brain volume of those being treated.

They noted that the longer an individual had been treated and the higher the dose of the medication, the greater the volume loss associated with the medication. They also highlighted the fact that the duration of symptomatic relapse was associated with decreases in total cerebral volume. The number of relapses a person had didn't affect brain volume.

If symptomatic relapse affects brain volume, but the number of relapses doesn't affect brain volume, couldn't this be chalked completely up to the treatment? Over time, it is known that people become tolerant of their antipsychotics, and their brain changes as a result of treatment. Could it not be that the antipsychotics are solely to blame for relapse and ultimately a majority of the brain volume loss? (Andreasen et al., 2013).

Fatigue

Hey, this thing called fatigue, it's not just the medications. What about the times you were not on medications? Or are those not on any medications at the moment? Fatigue exists because bipolar disorder is a brain disease, a disease of the brain. The brain controls your entire body, the very one organ that fails you in your ups and downs during bipolar disorder episodes and it affects your fatigue levels. Pushing yourself like a normal human being would is not the same when you have a mood disorder. Otherwise, pushing yourself too much will make you sick. Physically, you feel sick like a semi-truck drove by, nicked you only by a tad bit but left you spinning like the Tasmanian devil and left you with the full body aches of getting hit head-on.

> Okay, so what do I do? Remember, just to be you. You're you, recite this: **"I am me because I do and I will and that is I."**

Only you know your limits, does your body allow you to go for a healthy walk - you know you should be going on, or is it one of those days where everything is too bright, or too loud, or a combination of other physical symptoms? It's okay to take that day off. Read your body as much as you can to know your limits. Not being able to accept that you have a debilitating diagnosis, a chronic illness that affects you not just every other day, or some months, it's every single day of your life. You are not lesser than those without a mental health illness, you are braver and stronger to be able to endure the daily battles of bipolar disorder.

Hyperfocus

How many times do you experience problems with focusing and paying attention? A lot, but the same goes for the other side of focus. Periods of hyperfocus disrupt the lives of many people with bipolar disorder (seen as nearly a third of bipolar disorder patients have ADHD) (LaBouff, 2016).

It is not only focusing on one project but starting many single tasks or thoughts at once and trying to finish them but never reaching that goal. Anyone who gets locked into this period of hyperfocus can lose themselves for hours at a time. This is the reason why many people enjoy hypomania.

What makes people latch on to a specific topic?

> *"Latching onto a subject is not unique to people with ADHD or bipolar disorder. There is a concept called flow that most people experience. Flow is a groove. When a person is in flow, focus is heightened, creativity is high, ideas conglomerate seamlessly and one point of focus after another simply falls into place."* (LaBouff, 2016).

What's so wrong with latching onto a subject or a topic and becoming really intrigued with it? Nothing until it becomes a part of a person that makes it dysfunctional. When the rest of the world is ignored and only the subject or subjects matter than that is when it does more harm than good. Hours of sleep are lost, responsibilities that should exist are pushed aside, and it all becomes ultimately too much for a person.

Extreme Thoughts

Many people with bipolar disorder will experience moments of extreme emotion, these can vary from being depressed, not mad; being elated or really high up, not happy; paranoid or delusional, not suspicious; and many more where our thoughts jump to extreme conclusions and our brain cannot help that.

Not everyone always goes to the extreme end of thoughts, but they are often seen due to anxiety, distractibility, overreacting to specific situations- all extreme measures of emotions and thoughts that push people with bipolar disorder to create a catastrophic situation.

It is important to try to moderate the thoughts that flow within the bipolar mind and learn how to redirect them in a way that will not harm us or others. The basic beginning of redirecting the flow of negative extreme thoughts is to recognize them, not needlessly worry about them too much that it makes them come true, and to rest whenever possible because it becomes exhausted. It's okay.

Eleven

Managing a Mental Illness

Accept Medicated Help

Now, let's get to medications. It always goes back to this, sometimes, people, all they can manage is medications but not therapy. Some doctors suggest that a combination of both helps, but if you can't — reading material about medications, your mental illness, and learning about the side effects or how the medications will make you feel is helpful.

> *When you begin this journey, it can take a few months, or the trip can come back where it takes 2 years to a decade to figure out what medications work best for you. And when you do find the right cocktail, have in mind that your body changes and so does your*

environment, so why wouldn't your medications?

It can be based on the time of year it is that medication changes or tolerance creates another ripple in changing up to a different medication(s).

Stop Hiding

A big part of managing a mental illness is learning to stop hiding it under the covers. Very much like you have taken steps for medications to help you through this mental illness or some other alternative way to manage your internal battles with the lows and highs, you can also live a life worth living.

It is not about being able to hide well or mask any of what you have to deal with any mental health illness; it is about accepting that some days will be good and some days you have to take those days for yourself to not have your mental health illness become too overbearing.

There isn't a schedule either, so something such as mental health illnesses doesn't just change on certain days of the week or certain months here and there. It is a constant battle and struggles to manage or recover from episodes hourly, daily, weekly, monthly, etc. And there are days when even when mental illness is dragging you behind, you still go out and get through the day to try to make the best of it. That's you not surviving, but daily living the best you can for yourself.

Often, the stigma of the people around you can make you feel like it's hanging over your head constantly. You worry about how others may think about the days you need off from work

Managing a Mental Illness

or are anxious because meeting friends just do not line up quite right with what's chemically imbalanced with your mental health at the time. People do not know when you have had a struggle with getting out of bed, are having suicidal feelings or thoughts that are not planned for or hear or see things that are not really there just your brain chemically being a clown.

Very much like the person who has struggled with their heart and lack of oxygen pumping through their body to make walking from room to room a difficult task; the same is for those with mental health illnesses because no matter the illness your health is worth far more than trying to do too much. You know walking is healthy but if your heart can't keep up, then short walks inside the house are enough. You know walking is healthy but if your mind can't keep up, then short walks inside the house are enough. Do you see?

Everyone will have good days and bad days, remember this. Understanding that you have limits, it does not make you less of a person, realizing that you have those limits makes you a greater, healthier person for learning to care for yourself more. Self-care is important, you want to go out with friends, be mindful, drink a soft drink or water, and you can have a good time and not endanger your body when you know alcohol or coffee can disrupt your behavior. There will always be this part of you to want to please everyone or try to fit everything in but scheduled days of rest. Use that couch and watch your favorite film. It's important to remember that your health is worth far more than going out for the sake of others or trying to do too much.

Guilt is one of those lingering habits people with mental health illnesses hold on to. Let it go. Mental illness is hard work besides the other life work you have to do around you. Give yourself the needed breaks, and have a KitKat if it helps or a Snickers bar if you are *hangry*. Seriously, enjoy yourself, get that sweet/salty/fruity/nutty/crunchy/chewy treat, and do not think about what you should be doing as of now. And if those feelings of guilt want to drag you, express them. Talk to your close friends or family members who may understand, they will help you understand that this negative thinking is not helpful. Lean on friends, if they know you because you are honest with them and have to cancel because you can't be chatty that day, they'll understand because as friends go you should be mindful in returning the favor.

Twelve

Comorbidity

What is comorbidity?
This is a psychiatric term that refers to a situation in which an individual will have two or more psychiatric disorders that often occur simultaneously. An individual with bipolar disorder is very likely to meet the criteria for one or more additional disorders in the DSM-5. By this definition, 2 or more coexisting syndromes do not negate one another, that is they do not cancel each other out, nor paradoxically does this coexistence negate the potential for one to influence the course, outcome, and treatment response of the other.

Again, scientists do not know why, but having bipolar disorder appears to make you more vulnerable to anxiety disorders, alcoholism, substance abuse, bulimia, attention deficit disorder, and migraine headaches. It is important to take note, when treatment of bipolar disorder begins, it can also lead to improving the other conditions. Unfortunately, treating only the other conditions and not bipolar disorder, can also worsen the symptoms of bipolar disorder and trigger a manic episode.

There are many illnesses that coexist with bipolar disorder. Substance abuse is very common among people with bipolar disorder, this may be because many undiagnosed individuals affected by bipolar disorder treat their symptoms with alcohol or drugs. Substance abuse has shown to extend the symptoms or trigger bipolar disorder symptoms, leading to behavioral control problems associated with mania that can result in drinking excessively.

About two-thirds of bipolar disorder patients have a co-morbid condition; such conditions can worsen the outcome of bipolar disorder and also compromise its management. Also, there are very high rates of anxiety, impulse-control disorders, and drug and alcohol use comorbidity in individuals with bipolar disorder - however, this may be an overestimate (Parker, 2010). Most (95%) of the respondents with bipolar disorder in the National Comorbidity Survey met criteria for 3 or more lifetime psychiatric disorders. Overall, the presence of comorbidities in bipolar disorder has negative prognostic implications for psychological health and for medical well-being as well as longevity.

Therefore, the challenge in treating bipolar polar disorder comorbidities is to avoid exacerbating other elements within the comorbid symptom complex-especially the core mood disturbance. Moreover, there are psychiatric disorders that are often confused with bipolar disorder, they are the following:

- Attention-deficit/hyperactivity disorder (ADHD)

Comorbidity

- Borderline personality disorder
- Cyclothymic personality disorder
- Schizophrenia or schizoaffective disorder
- Recurrent major depressive disorder
- Anxiety disorders
- Substance- or Medication-induced mood disorder

Thirteen

References

- Abdel Hamid AAL, Nasreldin M, Gohar SM, Saleh AA, Tarek M. Sexual and Religious Obsessions in Relation to Suicidal Ideation in Bipolar Disorder. *Suicide Life Threat Behav.* 2019;49(6):1552-1559. doi:10.1111/sltb.12540
- Andreasen, N. C., Liu, D., Ziebell, S., Vora, A., & Ho, B. C. (2013). Relapse duration, treatment intensity, and brain tissue loss in schizophrenia: a prospective longitudinal MRI study. *The American journal of psychiatry, 170*(6), 609–615. https://doi.org/10.1176/appi.ajp.2013.12050674
- Bipolar disorder. (2017).https://www.nami.org/About-Mental-Illness/Mental-Health-Conditions/Bipolar-Disorder
- Bipolar disorder. (2018).https://www.nimh.nih.gov/health/publications/bipolar-disorder

References

- Bipolar disorder. (2020).https://www.nimh.nih.gov/health/topics/bipolar-disorder
- Bipolar disorder. (2021).https://medlineplus.gov/bipolardisorder.html
- Bipolar disorder. (2022).https://www.mind.org.uk/information-support/types-of-mental-health-problems/bipolar-disorder/causes-of-bipolar/
- Coello, K., et al. (2019). Metabolic profile in patients with newly diagnosed bipolar disorder and their unaffected first-degree relatives.https://journalbipolardisorders.springeropen.com/articles/10.1186/s40345-019-0142-3
- Cook CC. Religious psychopathology: The prevalence of religious content of delusions and hallucinations in mental disorder. *Int J Soc Psychiatry*. 2015;61(4):404-25. doi:10.1177/0020764015573089
- Dailey MW, Saadabadi A. Mania. [Updated 2021 Aug 6]. In: StatPearls [Internet]. Treasure Island (FL): StatPearls Publishing; 2022 Jan-. Available from: https://www.ncbi.nlm.nih.gov/books/NBK493168/
- Dunalska, A., et al. (2021). Comorbidity of bipolar disorder and autism spectrum disorder — review paper.http://www.psychiatriapolska.pl/21_6_1421.html
- (n.d.). DBSA - Depression and Bipolar Support Alliance. https://www.dbsalliance.org/pdfs/medication_charts/BPmedication_chart.pdf?msclkid=d5687ca4c5c111eca98a8ab1e0efe057
- Elsevier. (2020, February 4). Mood disorders on the genetic spectrum. ScienceDaily. Retrieved July 20, 2022 from www.sciencedaily.com/releases/2020/02/200204112538.htm
- Gaetano, R., et al. (2020). Impact of bipolar disorder and obsessive-compulsive disorder comorbidity on neu-

rocognitive profile: A mini-review.https://www.psychiatria-danubina.com/UserDocsImages/pdf/dnb_vol32_no3-4/dnb_vol32_no3-4_346.pdf
- Hossain, S., et al. (2019). Medical and psychiatric comorbidities in bipolar disorder: Insights from national inpatient population-based study. https://www.cureus.com/articles/23030-medical-and-psychiatric-comorbidities-in-bipolar-disorder-insights-from-national-inpatient-population-based-study
- LaBouff, L. (n.d.). *Bipolar disorder and ADHD: Hyperfocus.* Psych Central. https://psychcentral.com/blog/bipolar-laid-bare/2016/10/bipolar-disorder-and-adhd-hyperfocus#1
- Mental health by the numbers. (2022).https://www.nami.org/mhstats
- Miklowitz, D. J. (2019). The bipolar disorder survival guide: What you and your family need to know (3rd ed.). Guilford Publications.
- NAMI. (2021). Survey finds treatment cost and stigma are major barriers to accessing care for mood disorders [Press release]. https://www.nami.org/Press-Media/Press-Releases/2021/Survey-Finds-Treatment-Cost-and-Stigma-Are-Major-Barriers-to-Accessing-Care-for-Mood-Disorders
- Nishiyama K, Sugishita M, Kurisaki H, Sakuta M (1998), Reversible memory disturbance and intelligence impairment induced by long-term anticholinergic therapy. Intern Med 37(6):514-518
- Rahman M, Nguyen H. Valproic Acid. [Updated 2021 Oct 11]. In: StatPearls [Internet]. Treasure Island (FL): StatPearls Publishing; 2022 Jan-. Available from: *https://w*

References

ww.ncbi.nlm.nih.gov/books/NBK559112/
- Schaub, R. T., Berghoefer, A., & Müller-Oerlinghausen, B. (2001). What do patients in a lithium outpatient clinic know about lithium therapy?. Journal of psychiatry & neuroscience : JPN, 26(4), 319–324.
- Stahl SM, Morrissette DA. Mixed mood states: Baffled, bewildered, befuddled and bemused. Bipolar Disord. 2019 Sep;21(6):560-561.
- Valproic acid (Oral route) side effects - Mayo Clinic. (2022, June 20). Mayo Clinic - Mayo Clinic. https://www.mayoclinic.org/drugs-supplements/valproic-acid-oral-route/side-effects/drg-20072931
- University of Cambridge. (2022, March 17). Lithium may decrease risk of developing dementia. ScienceDaily. Retrieved July 20, 2022 from www.sciencedaily.com/releases/2022/03/220317143710.htm
- University of Cambridge. (2021, December 23). Clues to treatment of schizophrenia and bipolar disorder found in a recently evolved region of the 'dark genome'. ScienceDaily. Retrieved July 20, 2022 from www.sciencedaily.com/releases/2021/12/211223225442.htm

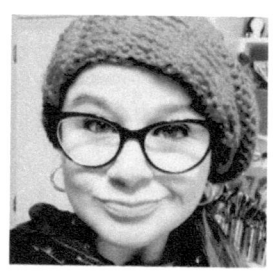

About the Author

Kimberly Jannice Brewer is a freelance artist, private mental health coach, wife, mother of two incredible human beings, working at home as a zookeeper for 7 box turtles, 6 baby box turtles, and three chickens (*thank you for the recent two eggs*), three dogs, three cats, three snakes, two red ear sliders, one musk turtle, goldfish and tadpoles, and two fat guinea pigs. She received her bachelor's from Southern New Hampshire University (*Summa Cum Laude*) and her master's from California Southern University (*Magna Cum Laude*), both degrees in Psychology. Born in Los Angeles, California, resides in Murfreesboro, Arkansas. Her dream home where she happily lives with her bipolar I self plus an infinite of other hobbies that come and go, of course.

You can connect with me on:
- https://twitter.com/KJBEccentricArt
- https://store.streamelements.com/kjbeccentricarts

Subscribe to my newsletter:
- https://kjbeccentricart.wordpress.com/blog

www.ingramcontent.com/pod-product-compliance
Lightning Source LLC
Chambersburg PA
CBHW031549210526
45464CB00003B/1228